The Practical Caregiver's Workbook: Strengthening the Patient-Caregiver Bond

By Sara M. Barton

Table of Contents

> **If we're smart,
> we ask ourselves
> one thing: "Can I
> do this better, for
> me and my loved
> one?"**

Introduction

Are you a family caregiver struggling to take care of a loved one? Do you feel like you are part of an invisible workforce that toils in the darkness, unseen by other human beings? Take heart. According to researchers, more than forty million family caregivers in the United States contribute more than thirty seven billion hours of time and energy each year to provide care for their loved ones. That's right. There are more than forty million other folks doing what you do. And many of us are finding the work as hard as you are. We are out there in the caregiver trenches every day and night, trying to do right by the people we love. It's not always easy, but we do the best that we can. If we're smart, we ask ourselves one thing: "Can I do this better, for me and my loved one?"

Any good relationship takes work. We constantly renegotiate the balance between the two of us. When one person is down, the common expectation is that the other person will offer support. It generally goes back and forth, to and from, so that no one is ever totally depleted. We give and expect to get our fair share in return. It's a cooperative relationship that nurtures both parties. There is a flow that goes back and forth in a complementary way; it's the duality of yin and yang. It is necessary to continually readjust the weight, the focus, the productivity, and shared power of the relationship. Normally, both parties usually are satisfied in the good times and able to manage frustrations during those times when things are not quite in sync.

But when someone is seriously ill or coping with a debilitating illness, that personal dynamic between the two of you changes. How do you navigate your way to the "new normal" and recover the equilibrium between you when one of you cannot function as before?

This workbook aims to assist you in troubleshooting some of the major issues you face as a caregiver, so that you and your loved one can better work together within the home care setting. You will have the opportunity to think about what you, as an individual, face in your caregiver role. The solution to every problem that stops you in your tracks must work for both of you, but because you are presumably healthier (and stronger), it falls on your shoulders to figure out the fixes for the problems you and your loved one are experiencing.

> **Sometimes it's difficult to admit that the need for a caregiver has skewed the balance we once shared.**

Chapter One: Something's Wrong

Recognize the Signs

The first step to fixing that something is to acknowledge that there is something wrong in the patient-caregiver relationship. The "something wrong" might be physical in nature, requiring new adaptations or adjustments. Or the problem might be complex and confusing because it's about the subtle changes in dynamics between patient and caregiver. Sometimes it's difficult to admit that the need for a caregiver has skewed the balance we once shared. When patients feel like a burden to their loved ones, that sense of guilt will create all kinds of emotional angst, and that angst will create fallout that will likely lead to more emotional upheaval. Unattended guilt can wreak havoc for family caregivers, causing serious and often unnecessary conflict. We need to recognize it for what it is, a trigger for negative reactions.

But it's not just patients who experience guilt over the need for a caregiver. Many caregivers feel guilty that they are healthier than their loved ones. Sometimes that distress can lead caregivers into dangerous behavior. If you feel remorse that you're healthy when your loved one isn't, you're headed in the wrong direction. To provide the best care for your loved one during a serious illness, it's important that you maintain your health to the best of your ability. Neglecting yourself imperils your loved one.

Like any good relationship, the existing connection between patient and caregiver must undergo routine maintenance. The bond is only as strong as we make it. It's important for us to work together in a complimentary way. Patients need to have a say in the kind of care given and caregivers need to have a say in how that care impacts their own lives.

There are some things that we must acknowledge. A seriously ill patient is on the losing end of good health. He or she may be frustrated that quality of life is being hampered by medical treatments, disability, or even a loss of function. A caregiver is sacrificing to help. He or she may feel a build-up of pressure and stress when the health of a loved one takes a turn for the worse.

Some caregivers seem to think they should take over the management of a loved one. They "know best what the patient needs." Unless your loved one has some medically diagnosed mental incapacity, he or she should be actively participating in the care decisions, both in the medical setting and at home. This ensures that the patient gets the best quality of life possible under the circumstances.

Who decides what the best course of action is? The definition of quality of life varies from person to person. Some patients want to keep working as long as possible during a serious illness. It helps them when they achieve their goals; that's what encourages them to believe in themselves and their inner strength. Other patients want to experience as little pain and hardship as possible. They want to live out their days in comfort and be as active as possible. Still others want to limit the information they have about their situation. They just want the basic explanation about their disease, treatment, and prognosis. They don't want to spend every day worrying about what is going on inside their bodies.

Every patient has a different personality and lifestyle. Every patient has different expectations about what is survivable and livable. That's why our goal as caregivers should be to support our loved ones and help them get what they decide that they need. It's about enabling them to do what matters to them, what makes living worthwhile under their specific situations and conditions.

So, let's assume you are willing and able to provide that kind of support. You accept the fact that you are part of a team of two people who hope to overcome the challenges that one of them faces. Here is your chance to think about what you can do to improve things between the two of you:

1. I know something is wrong with my loved one as a patient when he/she ____(fill in the blank)____.

2. I know something is wrong with me as a caregiver when I ____(fill in the blank)____.

If you answer this question quickly, you are probably in tune with your loved one's emotions and your own. If you are unable to fill in the blanks because nothing comes to mind, maybe you need a little bit of practice in recognizing the emotional impact that disease has on the relationship you have with your loved one. Be patient with yourself and keep at it.

Notes:

_____

_____

_____

_____

_____

_____

_____

_____

_____

_____

_____

_____

_____

_____

_____

_____

_____

_____

_____

_____

Strengthening the Patient-Caregiver Bond

Your loved one still needs to be engaged in doing what he or she loves during a serious illness.

Chapter Two: What's Broken?

The Big Picture Tells the Story

One of the biggest challenges for caregivers to meet is to make an accurate assessment what a loved one can and can't do. What are the physical limitations placed on your loved one by the health challenges? Is your mom unable to get around because she has COPD and can't catch her breath? Is your husband suffering from heart disease and at risk for a heart attack? Is your dad dealing with chronic and debilitating pain from the rheumatoid arthritis that keeps him sidelined? Is your wife going through cancer treatment that knocks her off her feet and upends the life you two share? You need to have realistic expectations of your loved one that are based on the physical realities of the health challenges.

Your loved one still needs to be engaged in doing what he or she loves during a serious illness. That's what provides quality of life during illness. So, how can you help with this?

As a caregiver, you are likely to come up against some difficult choices of your own over time. As a disease progresses, or when a loved one needs hands-on care due to serious physical limitations, the time you put into your caregiving will be significant. Where can you find adequate time, physical energy, and even financial wherewithal to provide it, while still being true to your own goals, hopes, and dreams?

It's quite common when you're under pressure as a caregiver to feel like you are flailing around in the ocean. Your loved one is counting on you to do the heavy lifting. You might find your anxiety level soaring as you wrack your brain to come up with solutions to fix the problems that are plaguing you and your loved one. What are the main sticking points for the patient-caregiver relationship at this moment?

The three most common complaints I hear from my loved one are:

1. ____(fill in the blank)____
2. ____(fill in the blank)____
3. ____(fill in the blank)____

The three biggest complaints I have are:

4. ____(fill in the blank)____
5. ____(fill in the blank)____
6. ____(fill in the blank)____

Unlike people without health challenges, a patient with a real need for a caregiver is already working overtime to survive. Just going through a day and night with limitations is exhausting. How do you help your loved one adjust to the "new normal"? Both of you need to recognize the changes that have come with the illness and accept that life is going to be different because of it.

But that doesn't mean you should just throw up your hands and surrender. When you strive to do right by your loved one and find solutions and adaptions for issues that interfere with quality of life, and you find ways to make peace with limitations that are what they are, you and your loved one can find your personal relationship is strengthened by the hardships.

Notes:

_____

_____

_____

_____

_____

_____

_____

_____

_____

_____

_____

_____

_____

_____

_____

_____

_____

_____

Strengthening the Patient-Caregiver Bond

_____

_____

> **How do we help patients with serious illnesses to feel connected to what matters to them here and now?**

Chapter Three: What Needs Fixing?

You Can't Fix What You Don't Know Is a Problem

There's some truth to that old joke, "Doctor, Doctor, it hurts when I do this...." Sometimes the answer really is: "Then don't do it." Other times, the answer is that you need to fix the problem. But how do you know what's really causing the trouble for you and your loved one?

Caregivers are often challenged by time and energy constraints. You are already facing a plethora of responsibilities. You're not only living your own life, you're also helping your loved one to live. When trouble surfaces, it often comes in the form of frustration. You might find yourself on the receiving end of an outburst and you have no idea what you did or said to trigger it. Or you might realize that your loved one is absolutely miserable, and you have no idea why. How do you navigate through that emotional mine field to identify the culprit?

Patients who are frustrated are often times angry or disappointed with their own bodies. I've had many patients with serious illnesses tell me over the years that they felt like their bodies let them down by allowing illness to ruin their lives. No one wittingly invites a disease to invade the body. These things happen to anyone and everyone. Is it fair? No. But it happens, and when it happens, we must deal with the result.

And sometimes caregivers have unrealistic expectations of their own. Believe it or not, I've had patients share horror stories of how spouses and family members blamed them for getting cancer. Some of my friends have been asked what their prognosis is and how long people can expect them to live. It's akin to having people measure you for a casket the minute you get a diagnosis.

The truth is that no one ever really knows how long we will live. People I thought would heal have passed away. People I expected to succumb to the ravages of their disease have survived it. I learned early on that no one can really know for certain what will happen. We can guess. We can hope. We can wonder. But even when a life-threatening or life-limiting illness wreaks havoc with a loved one, life goes on. How do we help patients with serious illnesses to feel connected to what matters to them here and now? What do you know about your loved one's views on the subject? Let's find out:

The three biggest obstacles that prevent my loved one from living the life he or she wants to have while going through this illness are:

1. ____(fill in the blank)____
2. ____(fill in the blank)____
3. ____(fill in the blank)____

The three biggest obstacles that prevent me from living the life I want to have while I am a caregiver are:

4. ____(fill in the blank)____
5. ____(fill in the blank)____
6. ____(fill in the blank)____

Does that insight you just demonstrated help you to focus on parts of your lives that can be improved? Are there ways you can navigate around the obstacles, or shrink them, even if you can't completely eliminate them? Sometimes patients perceived the smallest effort to be monumental. It means you care. It means you are thinking of your loved one.

It means that you are willing to think outside the box to get things done. With that successful gesture, you can inspire hope. Not everything that happens will always cause distress to your loved one. The more you get past the challenges, the easier it is for both of you to believe life can be better than it is at this moment.

Notes:

_____

_____

_____

_____

_____

_____

_____

_____

_____

_____

_____

_____

_____

_____

_____

_____

_____

_____

_____

Strengthening the Patient-Caregiver Bond

_____

_____

_____

_____

_____

_____

_____

_____

_____

_____

_____

_____

_____

_____

_____

_____

_____

_____

_____

_____

_____

_____

_____

_____

_____

_____

Every patient has a different perspective on what is comforting.

Chapter Four: What Can't Be Fixed?
Some Things Just Are

Coming to terms with reality can be hard. Advanced disease is what it is. You can't make your loved one better. That's a bitter pill to swallow. But you can help him or her to feel better. Comfort care is critical to a positive outlook for patients. What provides relief? It could be anything from a heat pack or cold pack to a gentle massage by a trained masseuse who understands how sore muscles are from being stuck in a hospital bed all day and night. It could be a ride in the car, just to escape for a little while. Every patient has a different perspective on what is comforting. It's important to know what will work for your loved one.

You also can't erase the impact that your loved one's situation has on your own life. That's not really going to change as long as your loved one needs a caregiver. How will you deal with this stress over time? What will you do if and when things get worse? All these worries and concerns can overwhelm the best of us. When we look at the big picture, the challenges can feel insurmountable. It's like being asked to climb Mt. Everest in bare feet. Is it even doable? "It's all downhill from here."

The first thing to remember is that you can always do something. And something is almost always better than nothing. You might not be able to fix every problem, but there are probably things you can tweak to make it better. You can and should find ways to bring comfort and relief to your loved one. You can and should also treat yourself kindly, finding ways to nurture your own body, mind, and soul. These efforts will help you get through the difficult times, when life seems unbearable, and they will enable you to remain emotionally connected to your loved one in healthy ways.

The biggest problem for my loved one right now is __(fill in the blank)__.

Three things I can do to make the situation better for my loved one are:

1. ____(fill in the blank)____
2. ____(fill in the blank)____
3. ____(fill in the blank)____

My biggest problem as a caregiver right now is ____(fill in the blank)____.

Three things I can do to make the situation better for me are:

4. ____(fill in the blank)____
5. ____(fill in the blank)____
6. ____(fill in the blank)____

Every time that you take steps to improve what your loved one experiences, you are providing comfort. That's a positive thing to do, one that will foster good will and trust between you and your loved one. It's the ultimate way to provide support. You are sending a message that says: "I believe in you. I know that even with all these limitations, you can still be active and involved."

That's true about taking care of yourself, too. When you take the time to think about what you need, you're reminding yourself that you matter. Your loved one doesn't always have the energy and ability to do things for you the way he or she did before illness changed everything. It takes courage and confidence to be good to yourself when you're already feeling the pinch.

Strengthening the Patient-Caregiver Bond

Notes:

_____

_____

_____

_____

_____

_____

_____

_____

_____

_____

_____

_____

_____

_____

_____

_____

_____

_____

_____

_____

Sara M. Barton

_____

_____

_____

_____

_____

_____

_____

_____

_____

_____

_____

_____

_____

_____

_____

_____

_____

_____

_____

_____

_____
_____
_____
_____
_____
_____
_____
_____
_____
_____
_____
_____
_____
_____
_____
_____
_____
_____
_____
_____
_____
_____
_____
_____
_____

> **People who are in good health require less support than people who are ill.**

Chapter Five: What Can Be Adjusted?

A Reality Check Can Save You from the Danger Zone

In a normal relationship, you give, your loved one takes; your loved one gives, you take. There is balance and reciprocity.

That changes with when a loved one has a serious illness. People who are in good health require less support than people who are ill. It doesn't mean that you don't have real needs. That illness creates greater priorities in the relationship you share. You have two people with very different needs and varying amounts of energy. How do you accommodate both of you fairly?

You will notice I didn't say equally; I said fairly. There's a difference. If you expected your loved one to function as he or she did when health wasn't an issue, you would be sorely disappointed. The fact is that people with serious illness can't do what they did when they were healthy. No matter how you look at it, your loved one is going to require more of you than you will get in return. Fairness, as a concept, respects the unequal needs of one person in the relationship and doesn't keep score.

Sometimes it helps to think outside the box in a situation like this, as a means of rebalancing the relationship. Your loved one needs your help to survive. You need your loved one's cooperation while you provide care, so that you can continue also living your own life. It's still a team effort that has some reciprocity. Knowing that your loved one is supportive of your goals is reassuring.

If all your loved one did was take from you, without ever giving back, you would quickly be depleted. (In cases of dementia, this often seems to be the case until other people join the caregiver to provide care.) For you to do what is needed for the patient, your loved one must be a willing participant in his or her own care. That's why it is important for both of you to recognize that your loved one is still a giver. You've got to have a working partnership that recognizes not only your teamwork, but also your contributions as individuals. Besides cooperation, what else can your loved one give to you that you can recognize as valuable? Every little bit helps, whether it's picking up the tab for a meal or sharing an activity that you enjoy. Those little gestures tell you that you are still loved and appreciated are valuable.

Hospitals and trauma centers constantly use a triage strategy to assess the condition of patients and determine who has the most critical needs. The doctors respond to the most imperative cases first, and the person with the least serious medical issue gets moved to the bottom of the list. That's what you will often have to do that for your loved one and yourself. It's up to you to prioritize who gets the lion's share of the attention. If you're smart, you will seek the solutions that benefit both of you. When your loved one feels well enough, you may find yourself taking time away for your own projects and interests.

Whenever your loved one is frustrated by the effort to carry out a task, he or she is likely to waste valuable physical energy fretting about it. That could have consequences that negatively impact his or her health, which can then create unnecessary complications.

More importantly, it can waste your valuable time, energy, and resources as you work feverishly to quell the storm. You don't want to get bogged down in your own frustrations or stressed by the pressure you feel to do more than you are physically, mentally, or emotionally capable of doing. You need to understand what your loved one is looking at and what you yourself see on the task board.

You also need to appreciate why it's important for your loved one to continue to accomplish important tasks, even if it means you provide adequate assistance. Self-esteem is often the first thing to go when our loved ones become dependent on us for care. The more we can encourage and enable them to continue to be active, the better they will feel about themselves and what they are doing.

1. The one thing my loved one really wants to accomplish during this illness is ____(fill in the blank)____.

2. The thing keeping my loved one from succeeding is ____(fill in the blank)____.

3. One way I can help my loved one to achieve it is to ____(fill in the blank)____.

4. The one thing that I can't do is ____(fill in the blank)____ .

Help your loved one tackle one task on that "to do" list with realistic support. Knock out one obstacle that stands in the way of a sense of success. Problem-solving together can be a real bonding experience. When you work together to discover one solution that will get the job done, you're telling your loved one two things. You believe that he or she can still get things done, despite the illness, and you're invested in making that happen.

Your goal is not to do the work for your loved one. If you did that, it would be your accomplishment. Instead, you're looking for a way to enable your loved one to succeed, because that will encourage your loved one to take on another task on the "to do" list. That's a big part of the "quality of life" experience.

At the same time, you cannot put your own "to do" list away. You still need to function in meaningful ways and tackle challenges that matter to you. That's easier said than done when your loved one's care takes up so many hours in a week. It's important for you to create opportunities as time and energy allow.

1. The one thing I really need to accomplish for myself while I am a caregiver is ____(fill in the blank)____ .

2. The thing keeping me from succeeding is ____(fill in the blank)____.

3. The one thing I can do to help myself achieve it is ____(fill in the blank)____.

4. The one thing I can't do is ____(fill in the blank)____.

You may find yourself frustrated by the constant drag on your own schedule. Just when you're ready to launch that big project, or you need a chunk of uninterrupted time to focus on practical matters, like taxes or bills, your loved one has a crisis...or needs to go somewhere right away...or must have your help to take a shower.

All these activities don't have to occur on demand if you can plan out what you're going to do and when you're going to do it. Time management is a great caregiver tool for knocking back unnecessary problems and providing a schedule structure, to bring consistency and routine to home care. When your loved one stops seeing you only as a caregiver and begins to appreciate that you have needs too, it brings back some of the reciprocity you lost to the patient's illness. It rebalances the relationship in healthy ways, by allowing both of you to realize that life goes on, even with a serious illness.

It also helps to remind you and your loved one that things are not spinning out of control. You will likely have times where medical crises disrupt your lives, but if your lives are basically structured to accommodate both of your needs, it provides reassurance that this challenge is manageable. It's up to you to define "the new normal" as a functional lifestyle, one that you tweak and re-tweak, so that there is some regularity in schedules you keep and certainty in daily routines you follow, even if the illness causes chaos.

By identifying what your need is, what's holding you back from getting it done, what your loved one can do to help you get it done, and what your loved one can't do, you will come up with ways to work around the obstacles. You will also see that your loved one really does play a role in helping you. If you need an hour a day set aside, and you choose the time when your loved one normally rests, you are far more likely to get that hour without interruption. If you pick a time during the day when your loved one is most active and needs assistance, you are likely to find yourself constantly stopping to aid him or her.

Notes:

_____

_____

_____

_____

_____

_____

_____

_____

_____

_____

_____

_____

_____

_____

_____

_____

Sara M. Barton

_____
_____
_____
_____
_____
_____
_____
_____
_____
_____
_____
_____
_____
_____
_____
_____
_____
_____
_____
_____
_____
_____
_____

Strengthening the Patient-Caregiver Bond

Sara M. Barton

_____

_____

_____

_____

_____

You and your loved one have options the next time there is a problem.

Chapter Six: What Can Be Rebooted?

Updating and Restarting the Caregiver Relationship Means a Fresh Start

Sometimes patients and caregivers get stuck in what was said, who did what to whom, and many of the other common pitfalls of interpersonal relationships. Clearing the air is often a great way to reboot. If you know that your loved one was in pain when he said this or did that, does that change your perceptions about the hurt you experienced? Surely you understand that a patient who is suffering, who is fatigued, who is physically or emotionally miserable, might not show you the love or respect you feel is due when coping with significant pain, discomfort, or even confusion.

And by the same token, if you have, as a caregiver, been up for two straight days mopping up vomit or you've been run ragged, you might not display an endless amount of patience when your loved one hits you with yet another request for help.

It's easy to be calm and cooperative when things are going well. But when times are tough, patients and caregivers both struggle. As crises erupt and tensions disrupt the peace at home, things can go haywire. Uncontrolled physical pain or fatigue can cause a patient to speak harshly or lash out at a caregiver. Should we take this personally and retaliate, or should we recognize what is causing the problem and work to fix it? Should we forgive and forget, or wait until a quiet moment to reiterate that we're there to help and we need to work together when there is a problem? Respect is always a two-way street, but sometimes when people are genuinely in agony, that pain really does take center stage. There's a simple way to tell if you're being verbally abused or it's an unresolved pain issue. Is your loved one kind and respectful when the pain is adequately managed? That speaks volumes about why we need to focus on comfort and quality of life. It enables our loved ones to be themselves and keeps them safer and happier.

Sometimes patients have unrealistic expectations of us as caregivers. We often become so adept at anticipating the needs of our loved ones and recognizing their issues, that when we don't recognize a new symptom or side effect, it seems like we've let them down. Disappointment and a sense of betrayal can make the home situation dismal and our loved ones desperate.

And conversely, as caregivers, we don't always appreciate how hard our loved ones work at surviving an illness. We're not the ones trying to get from Point A to Point B on damaged bodies that don't obey our commands. We're not the ones dealing with the side effects of harsh medications or the limitations placed on our activities by a seemingly endless stream of complications.

Some caregivers, when they get frustrated enough, might decide to run a patient's life by dictating what the patient can and can't do. We should never lose track of the fact that this is a working partnership. There must be cooperation on both sides in adequate functionality in home care. Rebooting the patient-caregiver relationship can go a long way towards repairing some of the damage done by caregivers and patients who are struggling under tremendous stress.

But as you work toward healing those emotional bruises, also take the time to come up with a proactive plan. Know that you can, with some practice, avoid some of the emotional outbursts by having a strategy in place.

What steps can I take to defuse the tension when I am exhausted and unable to think clearly?

1. ____(fill in the blank)____
2. ____(fill in the blank)____
3. ____(fill in the blank)____
4. ____(fill in the blank)____

When we are at odds, what can my loved one do to help me understand his or her situation better?

5. ____(fill in the blank)____
6. ____(fill in the blank)____
7. ____(fill in the blank)____
8. ____(fill in the blank)____

When you look at those eight answers, you should recognize something important. The weight is not all on your shoulders. It's a two-person solution. You and your loved one have options the next time there is a problem.

There really are times when the best solution is not to argue, but to step away and get some perspective on the situation. When the tension is overwhelming and each of us is rattled by the intensity of our feelings, it's important to take a step back and look at the big picture. Not everyone will see the same thing, and that's okay. We all have our own limits on what we can tolerate and how we can tolerate things. Caregivers who are frustrated with the limits on their own lives are likely to want to flee the scene. Patients who are fearful of new symptoms may be overwhelmed with the idea that dying.

Unlike "normal" relationships between family members, illness really does push us in very different ways in terms of dynamics. There is often a lot of fear in play when we are caring for a loved one. There's also a lot of fear in play for the patient with a serious illness. We're on edge because we're scared. We don't know how it will all play out or what will come next. You may find, for that reason, that the ability to be flexible in your responses is important. In home care, you really do sometimes have to let go of the small stuff and appreciate the big stuff. You have this moment in time. Tomorrow is promised to no one. Make today the best it can be.

The more mindful you are about how you communicate with each other, the better able you will be to avoid real damage. Even when a loved one is seriously ill, he or she can still help us to provide care by seeing us as human beings.

Sometimes, if we're very good at managing our "to do" lists, our loved ones don't see us as busy. They sometimes forget we're not "on the clock" all the time. There are times that we caregivers need to separate ourselves from our loved one. We do need "me time", but sometimes the only way to get it is to make sure our loved ones understand it's a necessity for us. We're not running away from them. We're not abandoning them. We're making sure that we get our own needs met, so that we can continue to be good caregivers when they need us the most.

Strengthening the Patient-Caregiver Bond

Notes:

_____

_____

_____

_____

_____

_____

_____

_____

_____

_____

_____

_____

_____

_____

_____

_____

_____

_____

_____

_____

Sara M. Barton

_____

_____

_____

_____

_____

_____

_____

_____

_____

_____

_____

_____

_____

_____

_____

_____

_____

_____

_____

_____

Strengthening the Patient-Caregiver Bond

> **Having a true companion that you can trust is very comforting to a person under stress.**

Chapter Seven: What Should Be Recycled?

A Real Need Is Not Something to Throw Away

Very often when someone is seriously ill, patient and caregiver spend a lot of time in each other's company. One of the most important roles of a good caregiver is to be a companion for the patient. Having a true companion that you can trust is very comforting to a person under stress.

But there are times that patients have needs that we can't meet, no matter how hard we try. Maybe there's just no time available. Maybe we just don't have the skills to do the job. And yet it still needs to be done. How do we make that happen?

Maybe your loved one needs more socialization, or fears being too dependent on you for care, or wants the chance to engage in different activities. As caregivers, we want our loved ones to enjoy quality of life. We need to understand that we are not the end all, and be all, of our loved ones' lives. It's okay to invite others in, especially as our loved one's health requires more support.

What does my loved one need that I can't provide?

1. ____(fill in the blank)____

What are the options for getting that need met?

2. ____(fill in the blank)____

3. ____(fill in the blank)____

4. ____(fill in the blank)____

5. ____(fill in the blank)____

You are likely to find that you, too, have needs that your loved one can't meet. Should you only do those things that your loved one can do and wants to do? Do you feel guilty that you have a desire to engage in independent activities when your loved one is ill?

If you hold yourself back from engaging in activities you enjoy, you're missing out on a great opportunity to de-stress. Maybe you want to go for a long bike ride with a group, not just for the exercise, but also for the socialization.

Or you'd like to take a class at a local college. Figure out ways to engage in those independent activities.

What do I need that my loved one can't provide?

6. ____(fill in the blank)____

What are my options for getting that need met?

7. ____(fill in the blank)____

8. ____(fill in the blank)____

9. ____(fill in the blank)____

10. ____(fill in the blank)____

Would you feel better if you knew your loved one was doing something fun or meaningful while you are off doing your own thing, or would it bother you if your loved one had a good time without you? Unless you're tied at the hip, it's good for both of you to have separate experiences now and then. It gives you both new topics of conversation when you are together.

Some patients do feel abandoned by their caregivers when their caregivers take respite time. When you're stuck at home because of illness, it can be hard to be happy that someone else is going off to have fun. That's why it's important to make sure that when you're engaging in an independent activity, your loved one has the chance to do something enjoyable too. This is a great time to invite family and friends to share one-on-one time with your loved one.

Sara M. Barton

Notes:

_____

_____

_____

_____

_____

_____

_____

_____

_____

_____

_____

_____

_____

_____

_____

_____

_____

_____

_____

_____

Strengthening the Patient-Caregiver Bond

_____

_____

_____

_____

_____

_____

_____

_____

_____

_____

_____

_____

_____

_____

_____

_____

_____

_____

_____

_____

_____

_____

_____

> **The human heart learns to be resilient and resourceful when we give it the chance to grow.**

Chapter Eight: Hindsight

If We Could Do One Thing Over, What Would It Be?

Every patient and caregiver has at least one regret. Maybe we zigged when we should have zagged. Maybe we took the quick way home when we should have gone for the adventure. Maybe we wish we hadn't held back the depth and breadth of the love that fills our hearts when it could have done the most good.

Whatever our regrets are, we do still have time to go for at least one more thing and we should do it. The human heart learns to be resilient and resourceful when we give it the chance to grow. That's one opportunity that serious illness brings to caregiver and patient. We are constantly reminded that time is short, anything can happen in the blink of an eye, and while there is music, Cole Porter reminded us, we should dance.

1. If you could do one thing over with your loved one, what would it be? _____(fill in the blank)____

2. What would your first step be to make that happen? ____(fill in the blank)____

3. How would you explain it to your loved one? ____(fill in the blank)____

4. What would it take for you to see it through this time? ____(fill in the blank)____

5. How will you feel when you get it done? ____(fill in the blank)____

If you can see yourself making this do-over happen, it must be important to you. If you can picture the process of doing it, you can reach your goal. And if you can imagine that it feels good to complete it, you really should go for it. These are the moments that make memories, the memories that keep us company when times are tough.

Notes:

_____

_____

_____

_____

_____

_____

_____

_____

_____

_____

_____

_____

_____

_____

_____

_____

_____

_____

_____

_____

_____

Strengthening the Patient-Caregiver Bond

_____

_____

_____

_____

_____

_____

_____

_____

_____

_____

_____

_____

_____

_____

_____

_____

_____

_____

_____

_____

_____

_____

_____

Sara M. Barton

Don't be afraid to celebrate the little victories you share.

Chapter Nine: What Has Been Improved?

We've Solved These Problems Together

Taking stock of the patient-caregiver relationship is important for several reasons. You need to know that you've overcome obstacles. You also need to know that as a result, you and your loved one are stronger together. Don't be afraid to appreciate the hard work the two of you have undertaken. Don't be afraid to celebrate the little victories you share. I've met a lot of caregivers and patients over the years, and one thing that really stands out for me is that once you've walked in these shoes, you have a much greater appreciation for the toll that disease can take on patients and their families. You also are likely to have a much broader understanding of how amazing and resilient human beings can learn to be when they set their hearts, minds, and bodies to it. The impossible often becomes possible because a patient has the courage to become proactive in his or her care, assisted by a supportive caregiver.

What are the hardest tasks your loved one has taken on?

1. ____(fill in the blank)____
2. ____(fill in the blank)____
3. ____(fill in the blank)____
4. ____(fill in the blank)____
5. ____(fill in the blank)____

What has been the most satisfying achievement for your loved one during this difficult time?

6. ____(fill in the blank)____

What have you done for yourself that you didn't think was possible while you were a caregiver?

7. ____(fill in the blank)____
8. ____(fill in the blank)____
9.____(fill in the blank)____
10. ____(fill in the blank)____
11. ____(fill in the blank)____

70

What has been your most satisfying achievement during this difficult time?

12. ____(fill in the blank)____

When you recognize where you and your loved one were at the start of this debilitating illness, and where you are now, you will begin to appreciate what your little efforts to provide comfort and quality of life have brought to your loved one. You will also appreciate just how hard your loved one has worked to stay in the game. It hasn't been easy for either of you, but when you've weathered a bad storm, you begin to understand that you have real skills. Why not continue to build on them and improve them?

Notes:

_____

_____

_____

_____

_____

_____

_____

_____

_____

_____

_____

_____

_____

_____

_____

_____

_____

_____

Strengthening the Patient-Caregiver Bond

_____

_____

_____

_____

_____

_____

_____

_____

_____

_____

_____

_____

_____

_____

_____

_____

_____

_____

_____

_____

_____

_____

_____

_____

_____

_____
_____
_____
_____
_____
_____
_____
_____
_____
_____
_____
_____
_____
_____
_____
_____
_____
_____
_____

Loneliness can be tough when you're a patient, sitting by yourself hour after hour, alone with your anxiety and frustration.

Chapter Ten: Facing the Storm Together

How Has Our Caregiver-Patient Relationship Brought Us Closer Together?

The funny thing about being a caregiver or a patient is you learn quickly to appreciate decency, kindness, and comfort. Those long hours at the hospital or cancer center can take their toll. Things go wrong, orders get mixed up, emergencies call the doctors away. It's often one problem after another. Loneliness can be tough when you're a patient, sitting by yourself hour after hour, alone with your anxiety and frustration. Knowing that you are going through this process together builds bonds between patient and caregiver.

75

Some folks think it's easy to be a caregiver. You just take the patient to the doctor's, or you stop at the pharmacy to pick up the prescriptions. But when someone is very ill, a caregiver is often the lifeline for someone who feels like he or she is drowning in a sea of sorrow.

When you analyze the transformation of your relationship, you begin to see what an incredible journey it's been. You look back on the hardships and sacrifices in amazement, remembering how many times you wondered how you would get your loved one through it. You remember those scary moments when it felt like the floor dropped from beneath you. You remember the doubts, the times you thought you couldn't go on, and yet you did it. How would you fill in the blanks for these statements?

1. Before my loved one got sick, I thought his/her biggest strength was (fill in the blank); now I think it's ____(fill in the blank)____.

2. My biggest fear as a caregiver was that I would ____(fill in the blank)____.

3. The hardest day for me as a caregiver was when my loved one ____(fill in the blank)____.

4. The toughest lesson I learned about being a caregiver was ____(fill in the blank)____.

5. The best thing I got out of being a caregiver was ____(fill in the blank)____.

6. The biggest change in my loved one since he/she got sick is ____(fill in the blank)____.

7. If I could go back in time and give my caregiver self just one piece of advice, it would be ____(fill in the blank)____.

8. If I knew ____(fill in the blank)____, I wouldn't have been so scared as a caregiver.

9. The three most important skills for a caregiver to have are ____(fill in the blank)____, ____(fill in the blank)____, and ____(fill in the blank)____.

10. As an experienced caregiver, I could teach a course in how to ____(fill in the blank)____.

Those ten questions you just answered form a very important inventory for you as a human being and a caregiver. You probably still remember all the terrifying moments, the aggravations, the sadness, and the worrying you did. But you managed to get through it and, better still, you managed to learn something about your loved one as a person, and even something about yourself. When you look back, do you see just how big some of those struggles were? There are caregivers who don't fare as well as you did. Somewhere along the way, they stopped trying to make a difference and settled for doing the bare minimum. They thought that less work meant they had it easier. But as you look back on your role as a caregiver, can you honestly say you would do less for your loved one if you had the chance to do it over again? We caregivers grow smarter, wiser, and kinder as we strive to provide the best care for our loved ones, and as we expand our minds, hearts, and souls, we benefit. Be kind to your loved one and yourself. Build on the love you have created with every mindful act. That is quality of life. It's what makes life in a challenging world worth surviving.

Notes:

_____

_____

_____

_____

_____

_____

_____

_____

_____

_____

_____

_____

_____

_____

_____

_____

_____

_____

_____

_____

_____

_____

_____

_____

_____

_____

_____

_____

_____

_____

_____

_____

_____

_____

_____

_____

_____

_____

_____

_____

_____

_____

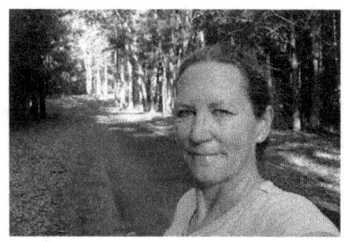

About the Author

I love to write, so you will find I am the author of several fast-paced cozy mysteries featuring lively characters like Scarlet Wilson. These tales are laced with humor and romance, but they are of the traditional style of cozy mysteries. The amateur sleuths typically reside in small towns and villages. The crime could take place in your neck of the woods. It could be your next-door neighbor who is found in a heap on the side of the road. It could be your dog that gets the first whiff of that cadaver and alerts you to its presence.

My determined crime solvers might not be trained to tackle big cases, but they do rub elbows with investigators who are used to dealing with wily criminals...and not exactly enthusiastic about having amateur sleuths along for the ride, even clever ones!

https://practicalcareguiverguides.org

https://smbarton.com

Facebook page:
https://www.facebook.com/sarabartonmysteries/

Twitter:
https://twitter.com/bartonmysteries

Cozy Mystery Series:

The Scarlet Wilson Mysteries revolve around innkeeper Scarlet Wilson and her knack for stumbling into murder most foul

The Gabby Grimm Fairy Tale Mysteries feature the good-hearted Vermont deputy who fights terrorists and criminals in Latimer Falls

The Off the Books Mysteries follow FBI Agent Henry Hartman as he takes on some unusual cases with help from beleaguered wife Sid and the hilarious Hartman ladies

Hybrid thrillers with cozy mystery elements:

The Cornwall & Company Mysteries chronicle "Marigold Flowers" and her life on the run as she escapes from ruthless contract killers with the help of Jefferson Cornwall

Stand Alone Books:

Frosted! -- a cozy culinary mystery